Straight Forward Medicare

THE CLEAR CONCISE BLUEPRINT FOR
SENIOR CITIZENS TURNING 65 OR OLDER

Roxanne Robertson

© 2022

COPYRIGHT

Straight Forward Medicare

By Roxanne Robertson

Copyright @2022 By Roxanne Robertson

All Rights Reserved.

The content contained within this book may not be reproduced, duplicated or transmitted without direct written permission from the author or the publisher.

Under no circumstances will any blame or legal responsibility be held against the publisher, or author, for any damages, reparation, or monetary loss due to the information contained within this book, either directly or indirectly.

Legal Notice:

This book is copyright protected. It is only for personal use. You cannot amend, distribute, sell, use, quote or paraphrase any part, or the content within this book, without the consent of the author or publisher.

Disclaimer Notice:

Please note the information contained within this document is for educational and entertainment purposes only. All effort has been executed to present accurate, up to date, reliable, complete information. No warranties of any kind are declared or implied. Readers acknowledge that the author is not engaging in the rendering of legal, financial, medical or professional advice. The content within this book has been derived from various sources.

Please consult a licensed professional before attempting any techniques outlined in this book.

By reading this document, the reader agrees that under no circumstances is the author responsible for any losses, direct or indirect, that are incurred because of the use of information contained within this document, including, but not limited to, errors, omissions, or inaccuracies.

ACKNOWLEDGMENTS:

I would be remiss if I didn't thank my son Mario Robertson for the constant encouragement, words of advice and expertise on the many particulars of getting my book published.

FORWARD

Make no mistake, attempting to understand Medicare in it's entirety can frustrate the best of us.

By finding this book, you have done yourself a tremendous favor as I have witnessed my mother help, coach, and guide thousands of senior citizens in the exact same position you are now.

Having a subject matter expert, who you can email or call at anytime for **free** with many moons of experience under her belt is a true blessing.

I trust the information you receive will immediately aid you on your journey, and I wish you all the best receiving the Health benefits you have payed taxes into your entire working life.

This book is for you to act as a quick reference resource, along with the ability to consult with a caring individual who makes this a seamless process.

-Mario Robertson

TABLE OF CONTENTS

- ACKNOWLEDGMENTS: 4
- FORWARD 5
- INTRODUCTION 1
- **CHAPTER 1** 5
  - ORIGINAL MEDICARE 5
  - PART A 6
  - PART B 10
  - PART C 13
  - PART D 14
  - PART E 14
- **CHAPTER 2** 16
  - MEDIGAP/MEDICARE SUPPLEMENT PLANS 16
- **CHAPTER 3** 22
  - MEDICARE ADVANTAGE PLANS 22
  - HMO'S 25
  - HMO-POS 26
  - PPO's 26
  - PFFS's 27
  - SPECIAL NEEDS PLANS 28
- **CHAPTER 4** 31
  - PART D PRESCRIPTION PLANS 31
- **CHAPTER 5** 39
  - EMPLOYER PLANS AND MEDICARE 39
- **CHAPTER 6** 41
  - INTRODUCTION TO ENROLLMENT PERIODS 41
- **CHAPTER 7** 50
  - WHICH PLAN SHOULD I CHOOSE? 50
- **CONCLUSION:** 56

Introduction

My goal in writing this book is that I hope it helps to bring you a clearer, concise understanding of Medicare which can be a very complex beast at times.

Working in the insurance industry sort of fell into my lap if you will. Call it a middle age crisis. I gave up a residential cleaning business and an Interior Design business to move to a small little town in N. Carolina to be near the beach on a whim. I had a job/career change in mind, and it wasn't insurance. I wanted to be a Family Readiness Officer for the Marine Corps as my son was a Marine and I was a very motivated Marine Mom as my son would say. Well, owning and operating a couple of businesses, one for over 16 years and the other for around 5 with a double major in design gets you nowhere in the Marine Corps workforce nor any other place in Jacksonville, NC for that matter. I even had a letter of recommendation from my son's Battalion Captain…no dice!

Meanwhile in Jacksonville, I had to obtain new car insurance and I asked the "agent" if they were hiring because jobs were few and far in between there. She responded in a very condescending way that "you have to be licensed" as if that was something I wasn't capable of doing. That got me to thinking a bit about the insurance industry, but not too much.

Needless to say, I tucked my tail between my legs and hauled myself back home, thank goodness I hadn't sold my house yet! I pulled a resume together and hit a few job fairs and low and behold I was soon called by a very popular, at that time, and not so large, now very large call center where you guessed it, I became licensed in multiple states for Life & Health as well as Property and Casualty insurance. Take that lady in NC!

I received superior training and had an amazing support team that taught me the ins and outs of Medicare. I became licensed in over 40 states and in the top 25% of agents in my division, often in the top 10. While call centers have a desire for large numbers in sales, I soon learned that I absolutely loved working with Seniors and I didn't want to just to sell them a plan to increase my numbers, but to help them and do what was best for their needs and not for mine. And when you lead the way with that type of attitude, the numbers come naturally. What I also learned was that a call center environment was not for me, and I wanted to venture out on my own. I have 9 years of experience as an agent who specializes in Medicare and now have my own agency doing what I love. I don't have a fancy company name, my company is simply Roxanne Robertson Agency, LLC as I let my name speak for itself. I have a very loyal base of customers who have followed me and tell me that I am their agent for life as I always do what's best for them and they know they have excellent coverage and that I am readily available for any questions that may arise which is something you will not get from a large call center. I am appointed and represent multiple A-Rated carriers to offer my clients an array of choices.

The purpose of this book to give you a basic understanding of the different parts of Medicare and how they work in a clear and concise manner. Yes, you could simply order a Medicare & You book which will tell you relatively the same thing. However, have you ever read anything that comes from the government that is presented in a clear and concise manner? Exactly, let's move on.

If you don't have a basic understanding of healthcare and how it works, you may find that Medicare can be extremely confusing to grasp with all the different "Parts" that it contains. I want to help you obtain a better understanding of the basics and what you'll need to have for coverage that fits your needs and fully protects you. My ultimate goal with this book is to help you better understand not only the basics of Original Medicare but also Medicare Supplement Plans, Medicare Advantage Plans and how they work. I will briefly discuss specific enrollment periods as I feel that they are important to know. If you have a desire to learn all of the ins and outs of Medicare, you can find everything you need to know on www.medicare.gov Don't make the mistake of going to medicare.com, you'll be asked for your personal information and will have multiple agents calling you in one day from those aforementioned large call centers. And trust me, they don't stop at one call.

As an I agent, I personally recommend Medigap/Medicare Supplement plans for the most comprehensive coverage. Those plans, however, are not affordable for everyone and you may need to have a Medicare Advantage (MAPD) plan instead. As Medicare Advantage plans tend to have a bad name for themselves, I will explain them in as much detail as possible for your understanding so that you can feel confident in the choice that you make for your personal coverage. Medicare is not a one size fit's all type of coverage and just because one plan works for Susie or Bobby down the street does not mean that the same exact plan is a good fit for you! Unfortunately, it's just not that easy.

Now let's dive in…

CHAPTER 1

ORIGINAL MEDICARE

Medicare was introduced in July of 1965 as a means to provide senior citizens with basic health insurance after finding that it was incredibly difficult for anyone over the age of 65 to obtain private health insurance nor were they being well served in the employment-based group health coverage. More than 19 million individuals signed up for Medicare in its first year with the very first Medicare card being issued to President Truman.

You are eligible for Medicare after working 40 quarters in the United States which is equivalent to 10 years. The quarters worked do not have to be consecutive. You pay into the Medicare system with every single paycheck via FICA. FICA is short for Federal Insurance Contributions Act. Along with your contributions, your employer(s) contributed as well. How nice of them, right? These funds are disbursed into the Medicare Trust Fund and managed by the government. Additionally, you may qualify for Medicare if you are:

- Under 65 with certain disabilities
- Are an individual with Amyotrophic Lateral Sclerosis (ALS), which is often referred to as Lou Gehrig's Disease
- Individual with End Stage Renal Disease (ESRD)

There are many parts to Medicare which may seem a bit like alphabet soup if you don't understand them. Let's examine a little closer.

There are five Parts to Medicare. Those are Medicare Parts A, B, C, & D and now they have Part E. You are only required to take Parts A, B & D without being penalized. Many don't realize that Part C is not mandatory and is your Medicare via a Medicare Advantage Plan (MA). A Medicare Advantage Plan that includes Part D is called an MAPD.

If you choose to stay with Original Medicare only (highly discourage this), your Part D prescription drug benefits will be provided via a private health plan.

Part A

Part A is often referred to as Hospital Insurance Benefits; however, it will cover more than hospitalizations. First and foremost, you will qualify for Part A automatically when you turn 65 providing you have worked your forty quarters and you are a citizen or permanent resident of the United States for at least 5 years. You may have qualified for Part A because you have a disability, end stage renal disease (ESRD) or amyotrophic lateral sclerosis (ALS). If you are disabled, you will automatically receive Medicare benefits in the 25th month after receiving disability benefits. In addition, should you already receive Social Security or Railroad retirement benefits before turning 65, you will automatically be enrolled into Medicare Parts A & B.

Part A is **usually** premium free however, you can purchase Part A if you or your spouse did not work enough quarters. You will have a premium of either $274 or $499 each month depending on your individual situation.

You may apply for Medicare at the Social Security Office or online at https://www.ssa.gov/medicare/

What's Covered

Part A for *most* will not have a monthly premium. It however, is not free to use. Part A will cover with *limits and restrictions* the following:

- Inpatient Hospital Care including acute care hospitals, critical access hospitals, inpatient rehabilitation facilities and long-term care hospitals. Not to be confused with long-term skilled nursing facilities.
- Short Term Skilled Nursing Facility up to 100 days.
- Blood
- Hospice
- Mental Health Care

Seems basic and to the point, right? You may have noticed that italicized limits and restrictions above. You would think that if you are hospitalized and Part A says that it covers hospitalizations that everything during your stay will be covered. Unfortunately, it's not that simple.

Deductible

Part A has a deductible of $1,556 (subject to change annually) which can happen every benefit period. A benefit period is 60 days. So, for example:

Let's say you are hospitalized on July 1 and dismissed on July 3rd, then once again are readmitted to the hospital on September 15th. A full 60 days has passed, and you will once again be charged the deductible. This can happen up to 5 times per year if you unfortunately become a frequent flyer of the hospital.

CO-INSURANCE

Depending on the length of your hospital stay, you may have to pay a co-insurance.

- 0-60 days: $0 coinsurance per day
- 61-90 days: $389 coinsurance per day
- 91 or more days: $778 per day for each lifetime reserve day. These are days when Medicare Part A may cover your care after 90 days in the hospital. You get up to 60 reserve days in your lifetime.
- After all lifetime reserve days are used up, you are responsible for all costs.

These coinsurance amounts apply to inpatient hospital costs. The cost may be different for skilled nursing facility and long-term care hospitals.

Medicare will cover stays in a mental health hospital as well and you have a lifetime limit of 190 days.

Skilled Nursing cost sharing is as follows:

- Days 1-20: $0 for each benefit period as defined by Medicare

- Days 21-100: $194.50 coinsurance per day of each benefit period
- Days 101 and beyond: You pay all costs.

What's Not Covered

Many things are not covered by Part A such as all the creature comforts one takes for granted while in the hospital. The following is an example of things I personally would take for granted having been admitted to the hospital that aren't covered by Part A:

- Private Rooms. Unless you need to be quarantined or it's a medical necessity, you'll have to share a room for Part A to cover you.
- The first 3 units of blood if they must be purchased by the hospital. Donated blood will be covered.
- Those very stylish warm fuzzy socks with the little grippies on the bottom…not covered. Also, any personal care items such as razors, toiletries and such.
- Doctor's services. Those will be covered under Part B.
- Television and Telephone service. Yep, you may be billed separately for those services.

I don't know about you, but all of those items listed above seem pretty necessary to me if I am to be confined to a hospital bed. What about you?

Another example: Let's say you go to the ER because you're not feeling so well. They decide to admit you to the hospital under "observation status". This means you're in the hospital overnight, possibly up to three nights, but not considered an "inpatient", Part A doesn't cover that. So, as you can see, Medicare Part A has quite a few gaps.

PART B

The requirements for qualifying for Part B are the same as above for Part A. You may however choose to defer Part B if you have creditable coverage through an employer or spouse's employer plan. If you have creditable coverage and maintain that coverage until you apply for Part B, you will NOT be penalized for not taking Part B as soon as you turn 65. Upon leaving an employer group health plan, you will have up to 8 months to apply for Part B without penalty. For most individuals, Medicare Part B will be $170.10 per month (subject to change on an annual basis) and can be deducted directly from your monthly social security check if you have applied for those benefits. Medicare will typically want bill you on a quarterly basis if you are not drawing social security benefits yet, you may call Medicare and change to a monthly billing cycle.

Should you have a higher income bracket, you may have to pay a higher amount for Part B. This is called an Income Related Monthly Adjustment Amount (IRMAA). You can find the IRMAA information on Medicare's website according to your wage bracket. Medicare has a 2 year look back period. If you have a drastic change in your income, you have the right to file an appeal. Here is an example below:

TABLE A

Individual	Joint	Monthly Premium
$91,000-$114,000	$182,000 or less	$170.10
$91,000-$114,000	$182,000-$228,000	$238.10
$114,000-$142,000	$228,000-$284,000	$340.20
$142,000-$170,000	$284,000 - $340,000	$442.30
$170,000-$500,000	$340,000-$750,000	$544.30
>$500,000	>$750,000	$578.30

LATE ENROLLMENT PENALTY (LEP)

You should note that should you fail to enroll into Part B and don't have creditable coverage through an employer or spouse's employer, you will be charged a late enrollment penalty. It is 10% for each year that you should have enrolled and did not. You also will only have a certain time per year to enroll into Part B once you are outside of your Open Enrollment period. This is called the General Enrollment Period. (GEP).

Part B will have an annual deductible. Right now, that deductible is $233 and is also subject to change on a yearly basis. What this means is that you will pay the first $233 out of pocket before your Medicare Part B benefit kicks in. Once that deductible has been met, it becomes an 80/20 plan. Medicare will pay the first 80%

and you will be left responsible for a 20% co-insurance for all medical services excluding your annual Wellness Checkup and certain preventative services such as flu and pneumonia shots, diabetes screenings, colonoscopies, etc.

Helpful Note:

It is important to know and take advantage of your "Annual Wellness Visit" with Medicare. This visit has a "zero" co-pay/co-insurance and if you are healthy and don't go to the doctor very often, this is your one opportunity per year to see a doctor with no co-pays.

WHAT'S COVERED

Part B will cover pretty much everything that is medically necessary and not covered under Part A. For example:

- Physicians' services including those received as a hospital inpatient
- Lab work and medically necessary tests
- Outpatient Surgery
- Emergency Room services
- Durable Medical Equipment and medical supplies
- Medications administered at your doctor's office such as infusions
- Ambulance Services

- Diabetes supplies such as lancets and test strips
- Bariatric Surgery for individuals who meet certain conditions related to morbid obesity.
- Chemotherapy

What's Not Covered

You should rarely encounter a medically medical service that isn't covered under Part B, however there are a few exceptions:

- Acupuncture
- Dental services
- Eye Exams and glasses
- Cosmetic Surgery
- Hearing Aids
- Routine Foot Care (critical for diabetes patients)
- Long Term Care

It is important to note that if you have a disease or condition of the eye such as glaucoma or cataracts, you will be covered under Part B medical services needed to treat these ailments.

Part C

Part C is a Medicare Advantage Plan. A Medicare Advantage Plan will combine the benefits of Medicare Parts A, B & sometimes D. Simply put, it is your Medicare managed by a private insurance carrier in the form of an HMO, PPO or PFFS. You will no longer used your original Medicare card; you will use the card provided by your private insurance carrier. You will show this card for all of your medical and pharmaceutical services. You will **NOT** lose any of your Medicare benefits by enrolling into one of these plans as you may have heard, you may gain additional benefits that Original Medicare does not cover. There is a huge stigma around these plans and individuals are told they "Lose" their Medicare benefits when they take one of these plans, and that simply is not true! We will go into these with plans with quite a bit more detail later in the book.

Part D

Part D, pure and simple is your prescription drug coverage. That is the only purpose it serves. It will not cover the cost of your medications in full. You can expect to pay a monthly premium, have an annual deductible and pay co-pays/coinsurance for your medications. Those co-pays and deductibles will vary by plan. In 2022 the maximum deductible for a Part D plan is $485. If you enroll into a plan with a higher monthly premium, there is a possibility that your deductible can be lower than the national average.

Part E

You most likely have not heard of Part E. I as an agent hadn't heard of Part E of Medicare until this year. They are now labeling Medicare Supplements/Medigap, Medicare cost plans and Pace program as Part E. I will go into these plans in more detail further in the book.

Now that we have the alphabet of Medicare down, let's explore the coverages that these plans provide.

Chapter 2

Medigap/Medicare Supplement Plans

They are one and the same, just called different names by different agents/carriers, etc. These plans supplement your original Medicare and cover the gaps. There are several different plan options, and the monthly premiums will vary significantly depending on the supplemental plan chosen and the state you live in. The most popular are Plans G and N. These plans are all standardized, meaning a Plan G is a Plan G regardless of the state you live in or the carrier you purchase the coverage from. The coverage will be identical. The purpose of these plans is to pay your Part A deductible and then cover the 20% that Medicare does not cover after you have met your Part B deductible of $233 (subject to change every year). A Medicare Supplement/Medigap Plan can be a life saver and certainly provide peace of mind as they provide some of the most comprehensive coverage in the world of Medicare. You will pay your Medicare Part B premium, Medigap premium as well as Part D premium if you choose this type of coverage. Generally, if you qualify for Medicaid, you aren't allowed to enroll into a Medigap plan and will need to choose an MAPD.

As I mentioned earlier, as an agent, I personally recommend a Medicare Supplement if your budget allows. The plans I recommend the most are Plan G and Plan N. Plan G will provide you with 100% coverage after you meet your Part B deductible.

With Plan N, you will have up to a $20 co-pay for a doctor's visit and a $50 co-pay for emergency room visits. Plan N also does not cover the Medicare Part B excess charges which is $15% above and beyond what Medicare allots for your procedure.

Example: Let's say you have a procedure that Medicare allots $10,000 for. Your physician charges excess charges, this means you will be billed $11,500 for that procedure. Medicare will pay 80% of the allotted $10,000 which is $8,000. Your Medigap Plan G will pay the rest assuming you have met your $233 deductible and you will pay nothing. Plan N will pay $2,000 after Medicare has paid their 80% of the $10,000, and you will be billed for the remaining $1,500.

Part B excess charges are charged by fewer than 5% nationwide. I always suggest that you ask your doctor before you decide about which supplement plan you take. There are also 8 states in which the excess charges do not apply. Those states are:

Connecticut

Massachusetts

Minnesota

New York

Ohio

Pennsylvania

Rhode Island

Vermont

If you decide to enroll into Plan N, you can always check with your physician ahead of time to see if they bill for excess charges.

If you, you have the option of paying the 15%, or changing doctor's and finding one that accepts what Medicare allows.

As you can see in the chart below, Plan G is the most comprehensive and you always know what your medical expenses will be, and that is basically your monthly premium and the Part B deductible. These plans are wonderful however, not affordable for everyone. If they are not affordable you will want to consider a Plan that provides less coverage or a Medicare Advantage Plan (MAPD). Please see the chart below for standardized coverages of Medicare Supplement plans. You will notice a Plan F in the chart below. If you obtain Medicare after January 1, 2020, you will not qualify for a Plan F, only individuals who obtained Medicare before that date are eligible for Plan F.

Moving forward, everyone will be responsible for their Part B deductible.

Benefit	Medicare Supplement Insurance (Medigap) plans									
	A	B	C	D	F*	G	K	L	M	N
Medicare Part A coinsurance and hospital costs (up to an additional 365 days after Medicare benefits are used)	100%	100%	100%	100%	100%	100%	100%	100%	100%	100%
Medicare Part B coinsurance or copayment	100%	100%	100%	100%	100%	100%	50%	75%	100%	100%**
Blood (first 3 pints)	100%	100%	100%	100%	100%	100%	50%	75%	100%	100%
Part A hospice care coinsurance or copayment	100%	100%	100%	100%	100%	100%	50%	75%	100%	100%
Skilled nursing facility care coinsurance			100%	100%	100%	100%	50%	75%	100%	100%
Part A deductible		100%	100%	100%	100%	100%	50%	75%	50%	100%
Part B deductible			100%		100%					
Part B excess charges					100%	100%				
Foreign travel emergency (up to plan limits)			80%	80%	80%	80%			80%	80%
							Out-of-pocket limit in 2018 $5,240	$2,620		

Plans K and L can be very affordable and give you the freedom of not being in a network-based plan like an HMO. You will have a co-insurance each time you obtain medical services with one of these plans. You should note that Original Medicare pays the first 80% and you are left with 20%. A Plan K will cover 50% of that 20% and Plan L will cover 75% of that 20%.

For example:

You receive a $200 bill for a doctor's visit which is the allowable amount that can be billed per Medicare guidelines. Medicare will pay the first 80% and you will have a $40 co-insurance left. Plan K will pay 50% of that or $20 and you will be responsible for the remaining $20. Likewise, Plan L will pay 75% of that $40 which is $30, and you will have a remaining balance of $10.

When you are in your Open Enrollment (OE) period which is 6 months before turning 65 (some plans limit to 90 days before your birth month), the month of and 5 months after turning 65, you will not have to answer any health questions and are guaranteed coverage. Once you are out of your OE period, you will have to pass underwriting to enroll into one of these plans.

You can enroll into a Medicare Supplement Plan anytime of the year, if you can pass underwriting. If you are declined, you can try more than one carrier depending on the reason why declined, some carriers are more lenient than others when it comes to medical underwriting. The agent you work with, hopefully me, should have a general knowledge of the health conditions which will prevent you from passing underwriting. If this is the case in your situation, you can enroll into a Medicare Advantage plan if you are in a valid enrollment period. Also, once you are enrolled into a Medigap plan, it's guaranteed renewable as long as you pay your premiums. Let's say, you try to apply to a different carrier(s) to lower your monthly premiums and are declined, you cannot be kicked off of your current plan. Just keep paying the premiums and you will keep your coverage. You can always change to a MAPD during the annual enrollment period should your premiums become not affordable.

When enrolled in Original Medicare and a Medicare Supplement/Medigap plan, you do not have a network of doctors. You may see any doctor anywhere in the United States, if they accept Medicare assignment. I have seen many times where a client has been diagnosed with cancer and they want to go to a specialty hospital such as M.D. Anderson or The Mayo Clinic. You can do so without any problem. This may not be the case with a Medicare Advantage Plan. Also, if you are a snowbird and live in multiple states each year, your plan will follow you.

You will be pleased to know that there aren't any dollar limitations on medical services provided by Medicare. You can receive as much care as needed, regardless of how much they may cost in any year over the rest of your lifetime.

Also, important to note, it is likely that you will have an annual rate increase every year on your anniversary date. This happens with all carriers in every state. There are a few states which are community rated and may go a year or two without any rate increases. Typically, once you have been in your supplement plan for 3 years or so, it is definitely to your benefit to see if there are any carriers that are offering the exact same coverage for a lower premium. You want to work with an agent, again such as myself who represents and is appointed with multiple carriers so that you have a variety of plans and carriers to choose from. An agent who is captive and only works with one carrier (a one trick pony) really won't have much to offer you and will downplay the fact that you can shop your supplemental plans as often as you like. In these situations, you will find that you are paying more than you need to. By year 3 or 4, it's quite common that you can save upwards of $30-50 if not more per month for the exact same coverage with a different carrier. I and any agent worth their salt will have a rule of thumb regarding supplemental plans: You should always be with an A-Rated carrier and be paying the lowest price available as the plans are standardized and are exactly the same from carrier to carrier.

You cannot be enrolled into a Medigap/Medicare Supplement plan and a Medicare Advantage plan at the same time. It is one or the other.

CHAPTER 3

MEDICARE ADVANTAGE PLANS

As I mentioned earlier, a Medicare Advantage plan is also referred to as Part C of Medicare. It is your Medicare Parts A, B & D combined into one plan and overseen by a private insurance carrier. You must continue to pay your Medicare Part B premium with these plans. If you qualify, you may have this premium covered by your state Medicaid office. An enrollee cannot be declined on a MAPD application because of pre-existing conditions. If you have ESRD, you may now qualify for a MA plan which is very helpful to many who have this health condition as of 2021. When I first started in the industry, an individual with ESRD was left with only Original Medicare for coverage. There are also Chronic Special Needs Plans (C-SNPS) to help with some of the costs of dialysis. It is important to note that these plans are not available in all areas, mainly low population or rural areas.

It is also possible to get a Medicare Advantage plan without prescription coverage; however, you want to be careful with this because you need Part D coverage and will be penalized for not having it. There are some prescriptions plans that are considered creditable coverage outside of Part D such as VA coverage. You will not receive a penalty if you have VA coverage and choose to enroll into a Part D plan later. You also may NOT enroll into a Medicare Advantage and have a separate Part D plan unless you are in a PFFS or Cost Savings Plan.

Example: Let's say you choose an HMO or PPO plan that does not cover prescriptions and you enroll into a separate Part D plan. You will be disenrolled from your HMO or PPO plan and your enrollment period will have closed. Therefore, you will only have Medicare Parts A & B for your medical coverage and will be responsible for the 20%. If it's affordable for you, you do have the option of picking up a supplement. If supplements are not feasible, you will not be able to choose a Medicare Advantage plan until AEP unless you qualify for a Special Enrollment Period (SEP). More on enrollment periods later.

It is important to understand that all Medicare Advantage plans must cover at least what original Medicare covers and they all operate under the same guidelines. You ***will not*** lose any of your Medicare benefits should you choose an Advantage plan, you most likely will gain benefits. Many of them will offer some basic preventive dental and vision care, gym memberships, over the counter credits. (OTC's), podiatry care and much more. Medicare Advantage plans vary from state to state, county to county, and quite possibly zip code to zip code. So, if your sister two states over that lives in a heavily populated city tells you about this amazing MAPD where she has a zero premium and zero co-pays on her some of medications, don't get too excited. That same plan may not be available or will vary in coverage in your area especially if you live in a rural area.

Premiums will vary by plans as well. It is very possible to obtain a Zero premium MAPD in several counties across the United States. You may also have a Part B premium give back plan in your area, and this is very beneficial for seniors living on a fixed income. Unlike those dreaded commercials (yes, we agents detest them as well as they are very misleading) that seem to air every 15 minutes on every single channel and state very misleading details, ALL PLANS WILL NOT INCLUDE A PART B PREMIUM GIVE BACK, NOR ARE THOSE PLANS AVAILABLE IN EVERY AREA. In order to qualify for the full $170 Part B premium give back benefit, you must qualify for Medicaid.

In most cases, you will not have a medical deductible to meet before the plan's benefits take effect, you will have fixed co-pays for all services received in most plans. However, over the last year or two, I am starting to see a few plans implement a small deductible. The zero co-pays that those dreaded commercials also promise are possible for Primary Care visits, preventative services and Tier 1 & possibly Tier 2 medications. Again, I cannot reiterate this enough, all plans vary depending on where you live. Unlike Medicare Supplement plans, MAPD's are not standardized, and benefits will be different from plan to plan and are subject to change on an annual basis.

All Medicare Advantage plans do include a Maximum Out of Pocket (MOOP). This is not a deductible and not to be confused with a deductible. A MOOP is the most you will spend in a years' time under this plan for medical services. Once you have reached your MOOP, you will not be responsible for any further co-pays for the remainder of that year. Very few people reach their MOOP. Please note that if your plan includes Part D prescription coverage, your prescription co-pays will **NOT** count towards the MOOP, only your medical co-pays. Most MAPD plans will include Part D prescription coverage. Please check with your agent to insure you have this coverage.

Now, let's dig a bit deeper into the different types of Medicare Advantage plans.

HMO'S

An HMO plan is a Health Maintenance Organization. This means that you will have a primary care physician (PCP). This PCP will oversee your basic medical care. If the PCP deems it necessary for you to see a specialist, you will receive a referral in order to do so unless you are enrolled in an open access HMO. With most HMOs, if you **do not** obtain a referral from your PCP, you may not be covered for the care received by the specialist. You also must obtain medical care within the HMO's network. If you seek care outside of the network, you will be responsible for the full cost of the bill. In rural areas and special situations, the plan may reimburse you, if you need to seek the coverage of a specialist outside of the network. In certain situations, if there is not a specialist in your coverage area, the plan will allow you to see a doctor out of network so that you are not denied coverage. It is best to call and check with your plan first so that you don't receive any unexpected bills It is very important to understand that Medicare will NOT pay the first 80% of the care received outside of the network as the HMO is your Medicare overseen by the private insurance carrier and Medicare no longer pays, the plan which you have your plan through pays. **I cannot stress this enough!**

HMO plans will typically have the lowest co-pays and more of the added benefits.

HMO-POS

This is a Health Maintenance Organization with a Point of Service network, essentially a hybrid of an HMO and PPO. This plan follows the guidelines of a basic HMO with a designated PCP, with a more flexible network. It allows members to seek care outside of the traditional HMO network under certain situations. You may pay some additional fees for using the POS (out of network) option such as a possible deductible for only the POS services and or higher co-pays.

PPO's

A PPO plan is a Preferred Provider Organization. This means that you can typically see the doctors of your choice. You can go both in and out of network to seek medical care. You will most likely have higher co-pays or co-insurance when you seek care outside of the network and possibly a deductible. Your agent is required to provide you with a Summary of Benefit's so that you are knowledgeable about these deductibles and co-pays/co-insurances. It's very important that you ask your agent about these co-pays and thoroughly read the summary. It is usually in your best interest to seek care within the network to keep costs lower. You will find that more doctor's prefer PPOs over HMOs.

PPO's will have slightly higher co-pays with added benefits. You gain the freedom of not being restricted to a network.

NOTE: With all the above plans, they will most likely include Part D coverage. Should you find yourself enrolled into one of these plans without Part D coverage you can NOT enroll into a separate Part D plan.

PFFS's

These are Private Fee for Services plans. These plans differ in many ways from other MAPD's. A PFFS plan contracts with all Medicare participating providers that accept the plan's payment terms. You do not have to choose a PCP. A provider may at any time decide to no longer accept the plans terms and conditions. It is always advisable to call ahead before your doctor's appointment to ensure that they are still accepting the terms and conditions of the plan. You will find that you may not receive as many added benefits if any with a PFFS such as the dental and vision. You will also typically have higher co-pays with these plans. Some individuals don't mind the higher co-pays because they have a bit more freedom to seek out other providers.

Healthcare providers are allowed to include balance billing up to 15% of the Medicare rate if outlined in the plans terms and conditions.

You may enroll into a separate Part D plan if you choose a PFFS that does not have Part D coverage. This is the only MAPD plan in which you can have a separate Part D plan.

NOTE: If you are a dual eligible individual (Medicare and Medicaid) you should **NOT** enroll into a PFFS plan.

SPECIAL NEEDS PLANS

DUAL ELIGIBLE PLANS (D-SNP)

You must be enrolled into both Medicare and Medicaid to qualify for one of these plans. They can be either an HMO or PPO plan depending on what's available in your area. If you are Medicaid eligible, you will typically have zero co-pays for your medical services and reduced co-pays for your prescriptions. You might ask yourself, why would you need an additional MAPD? These plans will provide you with added benefits that Medicare and Medicaid do not cover such as enhanced dental and vision coverage, food card and a substantially larger OTC credits and sometimes transportation. Again, these plans vary from state to state and are not available in all areas.

CHRONIC SPECIAL NEEDS PLANS (C-SNP)

A special needs plan is a Medicare Advantage coordinated care plan. These are plans that cater to individuals with a chronic health condition such as diabetes, ESRD, COPD and heart conditions. Upon enrolling into one of these plans, you will be mailed a verification form. You will need to ensure that you get this form to your PCP in a timely manner for them to verify the health condition and get it back to the carrier within 30 days of enrolling into the plan or you will be disenrolled the following month. These plans tailor their benefits, provider choices and drug formularies to best meet the specific needs of the groups they serve. They will typically have lower co-pays for medications related to the health condition highlighted by that plan. These plans will also have enhanced benefits such as a direct contact with a coordinated care provider. This provider will help to ensure you are getting the care needed for your specific condition including but not limited to home health care, transportation to and from doctor's appointments and many other services. These plans can be very beneficial should you suffer from a chronic health condition. Again, these plans will vary from state to state and are not available in all areas.

INSTITUTIONALIZED SPECIAL NEEDS PLAN (I-SNP)

This is a plan designed to help those who are in a short-term nursing facility for longer than 90 days or if you are in a long-term nursing facility. You can change your plan anytime you are a resident in one of these facilities after your first 90 days and up to 63 days after being discharged. It is extremely important to verify that your nursing facility is in the plans network. This is crucial and is your agent's responsibility.

Special Needs plans are required to develop a "model of care" for their clients to address the health needs of their target population. Thus, you will be assigned a team member with expertise in ensuring that all of your needs are met with the ultimate goal of improved health and circumstances.

Cost Plans

These plans blend part of Original Medicare and Medicare Advantage plans. They are very similar to advantage plans with a little bit more flexibility. You must be entitled to Part A and enrolled into Part B to enroll in a cost plan. If you do not have Part A coverage and only have Part B, the cost plan will not provide Part A coverages. These plans are not very popular in most areas.

MEDICAL SAVINGS ACCOUNT (MSA) PLAN

This is a high deductible plan that is combined with a savings account used to pay for health care expenses. You may have had an HSA through your employer and these plans are based on the same concept. Medicare will contribute to the beneficiary's savings account. You pay your health care expenses from the savings account and then out of pocket until your deductible has been met. Once the deductible has been met, the plan will pay 100% for covered services.

These plans cover Part A and B benefits. You will need to enroll into a separate Part D plan.

These plans are not available everywhere; however, are slowly starting to become more popular.

Chapter 4

PART D PRESCRIPTION PLANS

These plans are designed to help you with your prescription costs only. There are no added benefits to these plans. You can expect to pay a monthly premium (unless you qualify for Full Extra Help or Medicaid). You will most likely have a deductible and then co-pays for your medications. The maximum deductible that can be applied to a Part D plan for 2022 is $485. This is subject to change from year to year. For most plans, this deductible only applies to certain Tiers of medications. Those are usually Tiers 3-5. Tiers 1 & 2 and possibly 6 are usually excluded from the deductible. Again, this will vary from plan to plan. The tiers are as follows:

Tier 1: Preferred Generic medications

Tier 2: Generic medications

Tier 3: Name Brand medications or generics treated as name brands.

Tier 4: Non preferred brand medications

Tier 5: Specialty medications

Tier 6: Medications that treat a specific condition usually found only on special needs plans. They usually have a very low if any co-pay and are usually excluded from the deductible as well.

It is very, very important to note that the formularies are not the same for all plans. A medication that is a Tier 2 on one plan can very easily be a Tier 4 on another. These plans must follow the guidelines that CMS puts forth. They do, however, have the flexibility to charge different premiums and place medications on differentiating tiers as mentioned above. It is extremely important that you provide your agent with a thorough and complete list of your medications so that they can research the proper Part D plan for you. You should never, ever randomly enroll into a Part D plan or MAPD plan for that matter without providing this list. As an agent, I have come across situations where the client will feel that they are providing too much information about their health and don't want to provide a prescription list. You will be doing a disservice to yourself for not providing this list. Also, if you ever run across an agent that does not ask you for this list, they are also doing you a disservice and you should seriously consider finding a different agent.   As mentioned earlier, all Part D plans cover MOST medications; however, there is not any one Part D plan that will cover EVERY medication.

If you run into a situation where you are placed on a medication after having enrolled into one of these plans, there a formulary exceptions available to you that will include a medication on that plans formulary for the year until you can choose a different plan during the Annual Enrollment Period (AEP). Your physician is the best source to help you with this plan. Note that typically if a plan offers a tiering exception for a medication, it will be covered under a Tier 4 co-pay/co-insurance. It is not guaranteed that a plan will grant you a formulary exception and, in this case, you will have to work with your physician to have him/her prescribe you a different medication in the same category that is on the plan's formulary. Often times, the carrier will want you to try step therapy. This is where you are prescribed a lower cost medication in the same category to see if it will work before granting you a formulary exception for a higher cost medication.

If you find that you have a medication that is on a Tier 4, you can also ask for a Tiering exception to see if the plan can help lower the co-pay that you have to pay for that medication. As an example, they will move a Tier 4 medication to a Tier 3 so that your co-pay is lower. You will have to apply for this exception on a yearly basis.

Late Enrollment Penalty

You might be thinking, I don't take any medications, or I take very few medications, why would I need a Part D plan? The purpose of these plans is to provide you with coverage just in case your health status should change, and you need to start taking medications or your medication list increases. Think of them like automobile insurance. You don't purchase auto insurance after you have an accident, you purchase it before to protect you just in case. In addition, you purchase a Part D plan to avoid having to pay a Late Enrollment Penalty (LEP). This is a penalty that the government imposes on you for not enrolling into a Part D plan during your Initial Enrollment Period (IEP). The penalty equates to 1% of the "national average cost" of a drug plan. The national average is $35. The penalty accrues every month until your Part D plan goes into effect. Please note, that you will **NOT** pay this penalty one time, you will pay this penalty every single month for the rest of your life, unless you qualify for Full Extra Help (FEH), more on that later.

You have 3 months before, the month you turn 65 and 3 months after to enroll. If you have not chosen a plan, the penalty starts the 63 days after your Initial Enrollment Period is over. If you have coverage through your or a spouse's employer, you will have 60 days before and 63 days after the loss of coverage to obtain a Part D plan without penalty. Should you retire and choose to wait the full 8 months before enrolling into Part B, you will have 60 days before Part B takes effect to enroll. Once Part B has started, you will not be able to enroll into a Part D plan unless you have an SEP or you can wait until AEP to enroll. There are very affordable Part D plans available and well worth it financially to take one and avoid any penalties. Not to mention, we never know what tomorrow may bring and you will have coverage should you need it.

Part D plans should be reviewed every single year as they often change on an annual basis. Your agent may find you a plan with cost savings that would require you to go to a different pharmacy. A pharmacy that may be a Preferred Retail Pharmacy on one plan, may be a Standard retail pharmacy on another plan and this can make a huge difference in what you pay especially if you have a lengthy list of medications.

Please note: While change may not be welcomed, if you are working with an agent who does their best to keep your prescription costs as low as possible each and every year, it is typically in your best interest to make that change although you obviously have the final say so.

CASE AND POINT:

If a plan change will save you a minimal amount, say $50-100 or so I will say, this plan will save you a small amount of dollars if you wish to change. If a plan change will save you say $300 or more per year, I am going to highly suggest that you make the recommended change. Depending on how many medications you take, it can take quite a bit of time to analyze the plans that will be the most cost effective for you, and we agents get paid very, very little to change a Part D Plan. You may find that many agents won't even offer this service on an annual basis.

I have a couple of clients each year that I suggested a Part D plan change to help them save money on prescriptions and they prefer to stay with their current plan to avoid a hassle. Well, it never fails come January and February I will get a few emails and calls that state, "hey, my prescriptions went up". Well yes ma'am/sir they did. If you recall, I advised you to make a change for the following year and you chose to stay in your current plan. Unfortunately, you do not have an enrollment period now and you will have to wait until the next annual enrollment period to make a change. These clients are usually not very happy about this, but there is little we as agents can do at that point. So, if you have an agent that you trust and this agent has not steered you in the wrong direction before, please trust your agent and make the change. It's for your benefit, not ours, trust me in this!

In a rare and I do mean very rare situation, clients may find that if they qualified for Medicaid or Full Extra Help, Medicare may automatically enroll them into a Part D plan that there don't want or were unaware of. In these cases, you will have an SEP to make a Part D or furthermore, an MAPD plan change multiple times a year.

Prescription Drug Plan Phases

There are 4 phases to a prescription drug plan. They are as follows:

Phase 1: **Annual deductible** - You will pay all your costs for your medications until your deductible has been met. Some plans will only make the deductible effective for Tiers 3-5. Tiers 1 & 2 are often excluded from the

Phase 2: **Initial Coverage Phase –** You pay a copay or coinsurance for covered medications until the Initial Coverage Limit is reached. Your co-pays/coinsurance will depend on the tier that your medications fall under as well as the individual co-pays set forth by the plan that you are enrolled in.

Phase 3: **Coverage Gap Phase –** The most dreaded and costly phase also referred to as the "donut hole". Not everyone will enter the coverage gap, it is based on the retail cost of your medications that you and your plan pay towards. If you are on very few, low-cost medications, you have no worries. The higher retail cost medications are what causes you to reach the donut hole. For 2022 once the retail cost of your medications reaches $4,430, you enter the coverage gap and will pay no more than 25% of the cost of prescriptions until your out-of-pocket spending is $7,050. At this point, you reach the catastrophic phase. There are some carriers that will provide a discount during the "donut hole" and this discount may only apply to certain" *applicable"* medications.

I know these numbers seem alarming and trust me, they are in some cases; however, the numbers have greatly improved. When I entered the industry, you were expected to pay 45% of the retail cost of medications during the coverage gap.

Your annual deductible, coinsurance and copayments count towards the coverage gap. The plan premium, pharmacy dispensing fee and what you pay for medications that aren't covered by your plan do not count toward the coverage gap.

Phase 4: **Catastrophic Phase** - Once you have spent $7,050 out of pocket also known as your TrOOP (true out of pocket threshold), you are out of the coverage gap and enter into the catastrophic phase. You will pay no more than $3.95 copay for generic (including brand drugs treated as generic) and a $9.85 copay for all other drugs or 5% coinsurance. Ironically, these are the same copays you will have if you have Full Extra Help. These numbers too are subject to change annually.

It will benefit you greatly to utilize your plans "Preferred Network Pharmacy" vs. a "Standard Retail Pharmacy". You will always have lower co-pays at a preferred pharmacy. The plans often have several pharmacies that will be in their network. If you live in a rural area, you may find that your choices are limited. Mail Order pharmacies are a great choice as well as you will have preferred network pricing via the plans mail order pharmacy.

FULL EXTRA HELP/PARTIAL EXTRA HELP

Full extra help is a program to help people with limited income and resources pay for prescription drug costs. If you qualify it may lower your plan premiums, the deductible goes away if you have full help and your medication co-pays are greatly reduced. Partial extra help will require you to pay a small portion of your deductible and your medications are reduced by 25%, 50%, or 75% depending on your individual situation. If you have Full Extra Help it nice to know that the "donut hole" will not apply to you. You will pay the same costs for your medications as long as you have Full Extra Help status.

Either way this is a great program and if you think you may qualify **you should apply**. You may apply for full extra help at:

http://ssa.gov/benefits/medicare/prescriptionhelp.html

Chapter 5

Employer Plans and Medicare

I can tell you that the most common questions I receive are from individuals who are turning 65 and not quite ready to retire and confused as to whether they can continue to keep their employer coverage. There isn't one easy answer to this as all employer plans are different.

Creditable coverage is the key to keeping your employer coverage. If your coverage is not considered creditable, you will need to take your Medicare Parts A & B. The Medicare Modernization ACT (MMA) requires employers to notify their employees once they become eligible for Medicare if their prescription drug coverage is creditable coverage. This means that the coverage is expected to be as good or better than the standard for Medicare prescription drug coverage. If you receive notification that your coverage is not creditable, you need to plan on enrolling into Part B & D of Medicare.

Employers with less than 20 employees typically do not offer employer coverage after you turn 65. You must plan on taking your Medicare Parts A, & B. You can continue to keep your employer's health plan if they offer it and Medicare will be primary and the employer provided insurance will become secondary. It typically is best policy to disenroll from the employer coverage and take a supplement and Part D or an MAPD plan.

Employers with more than 20 employees will most likely continue to offer employer coverage once you turn 65. If you choose to keep your employer coverage, you may defer your Part B coverage until you retire. You should still plan on enrolling into Part A as there isn't a cost if you have worked your 40 quarters/10 years during your lifetime. I often get the question of "Which should I choose?" I recommend that a cost comparison be ran to determine which coverage would be more comprehensive and cost effective, your employer coverage or Medicare. I can run these comparisons very easily; all you need to do is send me a current Summary of Benefits for your employer plan and what your monthly premium is. If your employer plan is the best option, I will let you know this. I am not the type of agent who will automatically want to enroll you into Medicare plans as that is not always the best option.

Should you keep your employer coverage and defer Part B, ideally you want to start the enrollment process 60-90 days before your last day of coverage which is usually the end of the month that you retire. Remember, as long as your prescription coverage is as good or better than Medicare's and your coverage is considered creditable, you will not be penalized for deferring Part B. You will have 8 months upon retiring to enroll into Part B, although I highly recommend you do so sooner as waiting the full 8 months will effect when you can and cannot enroll into a Part D or Medicare Advantage with prescription coverage plan. With a Medigap, you have 5 months of open enrollment, again without underwriting.

As no two employer plans are the exact same, it is always best to compare and plan ahead.

Chapter 6

INTRODUCTION TO ENROLLMENT PERIODS

There are several different enrollment periods when it comes to being able to choose a plan for Medicare. It is your agent's job to know these enrollment periods however, it is important that you have a basic understanding of these periods so that you don't miss out on getting a plan that you need. There are certain times of the year, depending on your specific situation in which you may or may not be able to make any changes. Let's review these enrollment periods.

INITIAL COVERAGE ELECTION PERIOD

There are two ways to qualify for this:

- Qualify by age, meaning turning 65. This period will last for 7 months. It will start 3 months before your entitlement to Medicare, the month you turn 65 and then 3 months after. You may make one enrollment choice. Once the plan starts, that ends your election period.

- Qualify by reason of disability. Upon having been deemed disabled, you must disabled for 24 months and upon the 25th month you will become eligible for Medicare automatically. This enrollment period will also last for 7 months. It will start 3 months before the 25th month of being disabled, the month of the 25th month and 3 months after. You may make one enrollment choice. Once the plan starts, that ends your election period

This initial enrollment period allows you to enroll into Original Medicare Parts A & B. You should also choose a Part D plan at this time, or you may experience a late enrollment penalty. You can obtain a Part D by enrolling into a standalone Part D or enrolling into a Medicare Advantage plan (MAPD) which includes Part D coverage. You have one choice to choose either a Part D or MAPD. Once chosen and the plan is in effect, you will have to wait until the Annual Enrollment Period to change this plan unless you later qualify for a Special Election Period (SEP). If you choose a standalone Part D plan, then you may want to consider a Medigap/Medicare Supplement plan to cover the 20%. If you become eligible for Medicare by reason of disability, all states are not required to offer Medicare Supplements to individuals under the age of 65. If they are offered, there may be limited availability and you can expect a much higher monthly premium. The average individual that I have helped with Medicare that is under 65 generally takes an MAPD until they turn 65, then we switch them to a supplement at that time.

Being new to Medicare Part B also begins your *Open Enrollment* period for Medigap/Medicare Supplement plans. Depending on the carrier you can place an application with a carrier 90-180 days in advance of turning 65, the month you turn 65 and 5 months after.

ANNUAL ENROLLMENT PERIOD

The annual enrollment period is October 15 through December 7th of each year. This is when you can make the following changes to your plans:

- Enroll into a Medicare Advantage Plan (MAPD
- Change MAPD's
- Change your Part D plan or drop prescription coverage
- Go back to Original Medicare and enroll into a Part D only plan
- Go back to Original Medicare and enroll into a Part D and Medigap plan. *Underwriting will apply.*

Many individuals think that this is the only time that they can re-shop their Medicare Supplement plan and this simply is not true. You can re-shop your Medicare supplement plan anytime you want. However, if you are out of your Open Enrollment period, you will have to pass medical underwriting.

During AEP, you may enroll into as many plans as you like. The last choice made prior to the end of the period (Dec 7 @11:59pm) will be the plan that becomes effective as of January 1 of the following year.

Open Enrollment Period (not to be confused with your initial Open Enrollment upon being new to Medicare)

This enrollment period runs from January 1 – March 31st of each year. You can make the following changes to your plans:

- Disenroll from a Medicare Advantage and enroll into a Part D only

- Make a one-time change to a different Medicare Advantage plan.

- Disenroll from a Medicare Advantage and enroll into a Part D only and a Medicare Supplement. *Underwriting will apply.*

GENERAL ENROLLMENT PERIOD

This period too runs from January 1 through March 31st of each year. This is when you could enroll into Part B of Medicare if you missed your initial election period. You may expect to have a late enrollment penalty and your Medicare Part B will not take effect until July 1 of the year you enrolled. You will have a onetime opportunity to enroll into a Part D plan if not already enrolled into one or a Medicare Advantage plan. These plans must be enrolled to before July 1st of that year. If you do not have these plans in place by July 1, you will have to wait until the Annual Election Period (AEP) to make a plan choice unless you qualify for a Special enrollment period (SEP).

You will also be able to enroll into a Medicare Supplement plan if you choose without going through underwriting.

INITIAL ELECTION PERIOD

If you deferred Part B because you decided to continue working after turning 65 or you have employer coverage via your spouse, you have a Special Election Period to enroll into Part B and then choose your plan or plans to go along with your Medicare Parts A & B. You have 8 months after losing employer group health coverage to enroll into Part B without a penalty. In regard to Part D plans or Medicare Advantage plans you have 60 days before your Part B starts to choose a plan that will coincide with your Part B coverage start date.

If you enroll into Part B 60 days before retiring, you will also have 60 days after Part B starts to enroll into your chosen plans that must start on the following month after enrollment.

There is a certain hierarchy to the different enrollment periods, and you may be in more than enrollment period at a time which is entirely possible. You do not need to worry about the hierarchy. If you work with a qualified agent, they will now which enrollment period to apply for on your applications.

SPECIAL ENROLLMENT PERIODS

There are many reasons that you can enter a Special Election Period. This election period usually means a life changing event has happened such as retiring, moving, living in a Skilled Nursing Facility or being released from incarceration. There may be FEMA related SEP's as well. This is a SEP is available for a very short period of time and you must have resided in an area where a natural disaster has occurred. You can make the following changes:

- As a result of moving, you can change your Part D plan or Medicare Advantage plan. (a move must include a change in zip codes) If you had a Medicare Advantage plan before moving, you may be considered Guarantee Issue for a Medicare Supplement. This is the only other way outside of Open Enrollment to obtain a Medicare Supplement without having to go through the underwriting process except for a handful of states that have their own specific rule that allows you a once per year option to change to a plan with the exact coverage you currently have or lower. You have 30 days before the move, the month of and 63 days after your move to change plans. Please note: a move does not create a special election period to change from one Medicare Supplement to another. As a reminder you can reshop your Medicare supplement anytime you wish if you are healthy enough to pass underwriting.

- Being released from incarceration will allow you to enroll into a Medicare Advantage or Part D plan. You have 63 days to make this choice.

- Having a 90 day stay or longer in a Skilled Nursing Facility or Nursing Home will allow you to change your Medicare Advantage Plan or Part D plan at any time. You will NOT qualify for a Medicare supplement if you are a current resident of one of the facilities.

- If you are enrolled into a MAPD, MA only or PDP plan that leaves the coverage area, you will have a SEP to choose and enroll into a new plan. This doesn't happen often, but if it does, you probably needed a new plan anyway. When this happens, it means that the plan was no longer meeting Medicare's guidelines and or they went bankrupt.

- If you live in a coverage area where there is a 5-star plan available, you may change to that plan one time per year.

- Involuntary loss of creditable drug coverage or employer coverage

- Becoming eligible for or losing Medicaid. You are eligible to change your plan once every quarter if you have Medicaid.

- Gaining or losing the Part D low-income subsidy referred to as Extra Help. You are eligible to change your plan once every quarter if you have Extra Help.

- Being diagnosed with a chronic illness such as diabetes, COPD or ESRD (end stage renal disease) if there is a Chronic Special Needs plan pertaining to your specific diagnosis available in your coverage area.

Note: If you have been deemed an "at-risk" individual for misuse or abuse of a frequently abused drug per the requirements for the drug management programs, you are no longer eligible for the quarterly SEP to change plans if you have Extra Help or Medicaid. You do have the right to appeal this decision.

The SEP rules stated below apply to Medicare Supplement plans only:

- Missouri has an annual enrollment period called the Anniversary Rule. This means you may change your plan to a like plan such as a Plan G or you may move down to a Plan N without any health questions and regardless of any pre-existing conditions. You may not move up in coverage from a Plan N or High Deductible G during this SEP. You would have to qualify for underwriting to move up in coverage.

- California, Idaho, Illinois, Oregon, and Nevada have an annual birthday rule. You may make a lateral change to the same plan regardless of pre-existing conditions. You can make this change with 30 days of your birthdate.

The reason why you would want to implement the latter of the two SEP's is if your premiums have gone up significantly and you may be able to move to a different carrier with lower premiums.

Disaster Relief Enrollment Period

If you live in an area where a natural disaster has occurred, CMS may work with your state at their discretion to offer a disaster relief enrollment period. These enrollment periods always have a specific date stamp attached to them and once that date has passed, you will have to wait until the next enrollment opens to choose a plan should you miss the date to enroll.

Medigap SEP

If you enrolled into a Medigap/Medicare Supplement plan as your initial coverage election and you decide to drop that plan to enroll into a MA/MAPD for the first time, you have 12 months from the start date to disenroll from your MA/MAPD and re-enroll into a Medicare Supplement plan. You will have guaranteed eligibility to rejoin the Medigap plan. You only have one opportunity to use this SEP.

There are many different timelines associated with each enrollment period or SEP. You need not be concerned with the timelines as your agent should be well adept and help you make an informed decision.

While enrolled into any plan that requires a monthly premium, should you fail to pay that premium, the plan sponsor may offer you a 60-day grace period to bring your premiums current. Should you fail to do so and are disenrolled from a plan, you DO NOT have an SEP to enroll into another plan as a result of having failed to pay your plans premiums.

Chapter 7

Which Plan Should I Choose?

I as an agent cannot make this decision for you. I can only inform you of your options and guide you. There is no right or wrong answer to this question.

I'll never forget a client I once spoke with. He was in the ICU for 10 days after having had quadruple bypass surgery. After all was said and done, and Medicare had paid their share, he still had over $150,000 in bills. The worst part was that he only had Original Medicare and there was nothing I could do for him as he wasn't in an enrollment period, nor could he pass underwriting for a Medicare Supplement. I did call this gentleman back during AEP and got him enrolled into a Medicare Advantage plan as he was again, not able to pass underwriting for a Medicare Supplement. He was so grateful to know that should he find himself in that predicament again, he at least had a maximum out of pocket in place (MOOP). We were both in tears by the end of that phone call.

Thus, being said, Medicare was NEVER meant to be your only coverage. There are too many gaps that leave you susceptible to very large bills and let's face it, when you retire you are generally on a fixed income. As I mentioned previously, I typically recommend a Medicare Supplement as it provides the most predictable coverage, and you always know what your monthly bills will be. Your Medicare premium + Medigap premium + Part D premium. If you choose Plan G, you have the annual deductible which again is the Medicare Part B deductible of $233 (subject to change annually) and then 100% coverage for anything medically necessary after that without being restricted to any networks.

I have many clients who tell me they are perfectly healthy and don't want to pay the premiums of a Medigap plan and they would rather choose a low or zero premium MAPD, then take a Medigap in a few years. This is perfectly fine as you have the Trial Right to join a Medigap plan within the first year without any health questions. After that, you must undergo medical underwriting. And let's face it, some of us find ourselves perfectly healthy today and, in the hospital, tomorrow with a life-threatening complication as tomorrow is never promised to us. So, you may have to keep a MAPD and not have the opportunity to enroll into Medigap. And there is nothing wrong with that at all, your coverage just won't be quite as comprehensive.

Many simply cannot afford a Medigap and therefore an MAPD is their only option. I assure you that you will still have excellent coverage however, your costs may be a bit unpredictable from month to month should you become a bit unhealthier. You will have very low or even zero premiums in most areas which is nice. However, you will have co-pays/coinsurance just about every time you use the plan. Your preventative screenings won't have co-pays and perhaps your PCP visit will have a zero co-pay. For all other services, you can expect to pay. So, if you find yourself needing an outpatient surgery, you will have a co-pay of a few hundred dollar or so. This is where your unpredictable charges come in. Also, you should note that MAPD plans may require prior authorizations for certain procedures, which for some people can be frustrating as the plan may require you try an alternative treatment first.

Example: Your PCP wants you to have a sleep study test for possible sleep apnea. Your plan may authorize an at home sleep study rather than a overnight sleep study at a medical facility. The results may not be as accurate if performed at home. Not to mention, you must wire yourself for sound and attempt to sleep after that. Speaking from a bit of experience here.

Some individuals know immediately what they want, and we get right to the enrollments. Other times, they need to sleep on it for a day or two before a decision is made. As an agent, I never push my clients to decide immediately as turning 65 and/or becoming eligible for Medicare is a life changing event. It is a lot to think about and you should never be rushed into making an immediate decision. If you are working with an agent that pushes you to make this decision the same day, you should find another agent, preferably me! This chart may help you make a choice should you take the Medicare Advantage route. Note that plans vary by state, county and zip codes. All plans may not be available in your coverage area.

MA/MAPD	HMO	HMO-POS	LPPO	RPPO
	These plans are network based and have coordinated care	Primarily coordinated care with a some out of network benefits	These plans will offer out of network access for freedom of choice	Regional PPO covers multiple states, usually found in rural areas.
What is it?	Health Maintenance organization (HMO) Must use network providers except in the case of an emergency, urgent care or dialysis.	An HMO with a few out of network benefits.	Preferred Provider Organization (PPO) Flexibility to see providers in and out of network. Out of network may be at a higher cost.	Same as a LPPO with a wider range of providers in multiple states, usually only available in rural areas or cities that border

				another state
Who would like it?	Consumers willing to use network providers for lower co-pays	Consumers willing to use network providers and willing to pay higher cost for limited out of network services	Members who prefer freedom of choice for their providers. Will pay less for in network services.	Members who live in rural areas with limited providers. Will pay less for in network services. Providers may be in various bordering states.

| How does it work? | Must get care from in network providers. Will be billed for the full amount for any out of network services | Mostly in network services with out of network availability for limited services. | Freedom of choice with lower co-pays for in network services. Ok with paying higher co-pays for out of network services | Same as LPPO with providers in multiple states. |

Conclusion:

Upon taking your Medicare, you will have it until end of life unless you move out of the country, or you stop paying your premiums. It is not a decision to be taken lightly when it comes to your coverage. You should never have to decide between paying your premiums or purchasing medication or food. Please run the numbers and make the decision that best fits you.

As I mentioned, I have been in the insurance industry for 9 years and I specialize in Medicare. I am currently licensed in over 40 states. I can also help with dental/vision, final expense, critical illness and life insurance. My specialty and passion is Medicare Insurance. I truly enjoy working with seniors and helping them navigate their options with Medicare. Sadly, there are so many shady agents out there only after a commission and that is the wrong reason to be in the insurance industry. I have often consulted with a potential client and let them know that a plan that I do NOT represent is a better option for them as that is the right thing to do.

My consultations are free, you may pick my brain at will.

I would love to work with you and be your reliable agent for life!

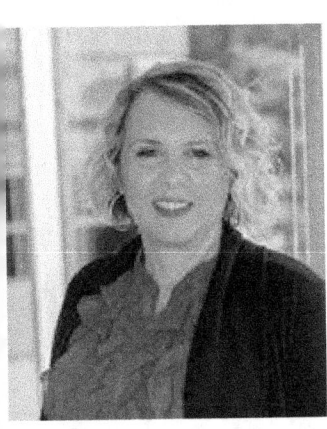

My contact information:

Email – roxanne@rragency.net

Phone – 913-593-1291

Facebook - https://www.facebook.com/rrobertsonagency

Instagram - https://www.instagram.com/themedicarelady2

LinkedIn – https://www.linkedin.com/in/roxanne-robertson-b5b1ab20/

www.ingramcontent.com/pod-product-compliance
Lightning Source LLC
Chambersburg PA
CBHW070318220526
45465CB00004B/1902